MY HAPPY CELLS
By Jill P. Boyce

Illustrated by
Cindy Lou Fancher

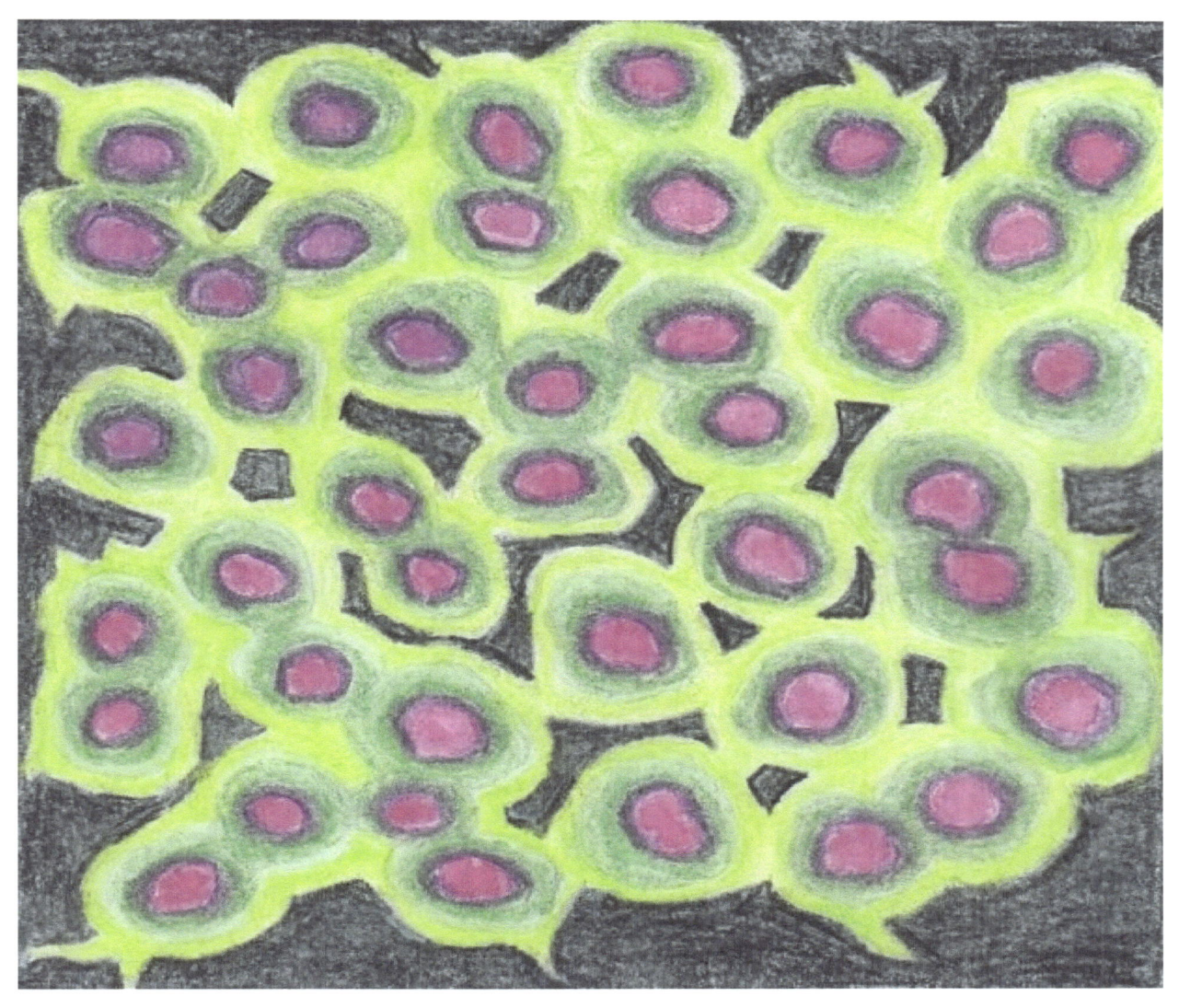

My body is made up of thousands of cells.

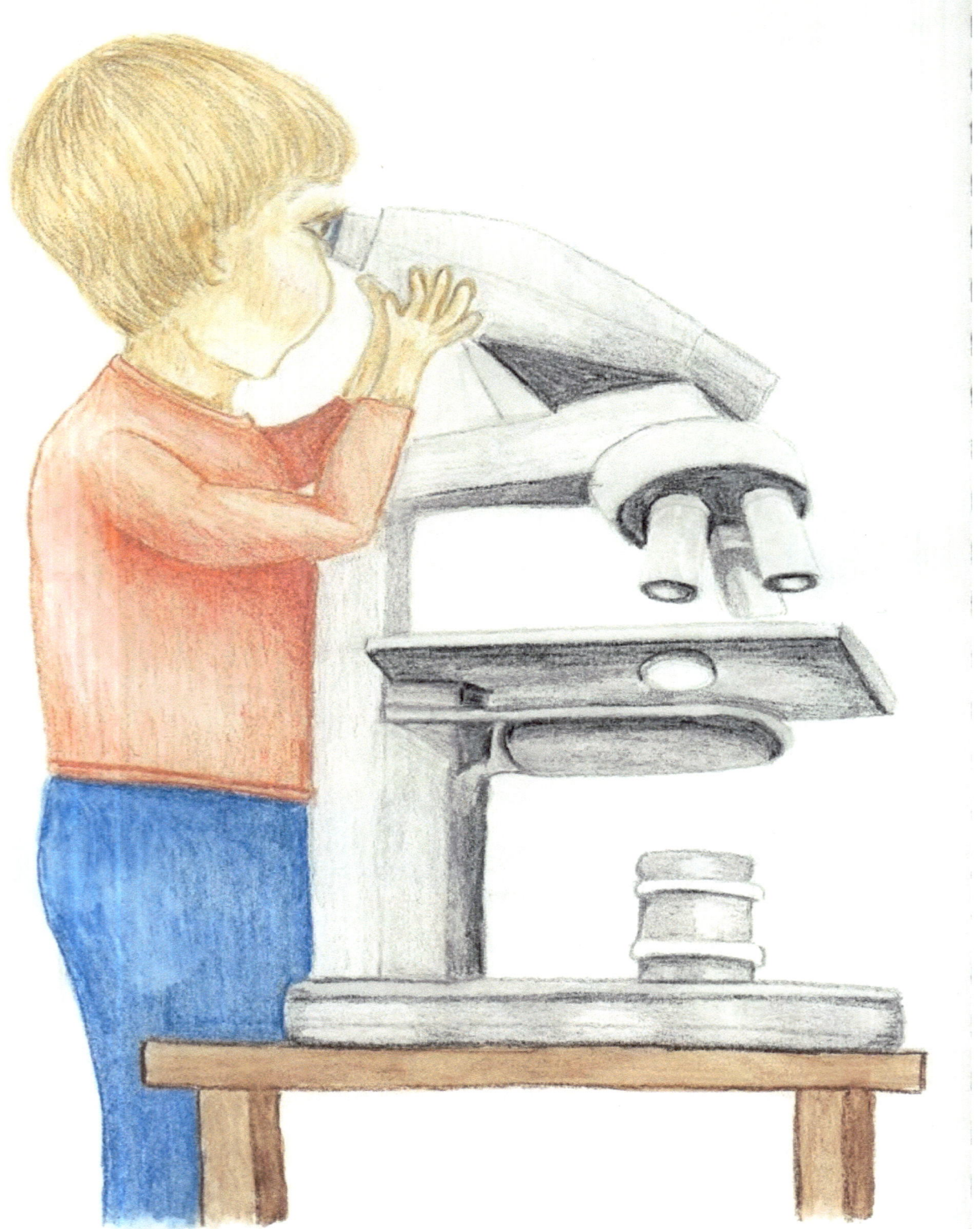

My cells are too small
to see, so if I want
to see what my cells
look like, I have to
look at them under
a microscope.

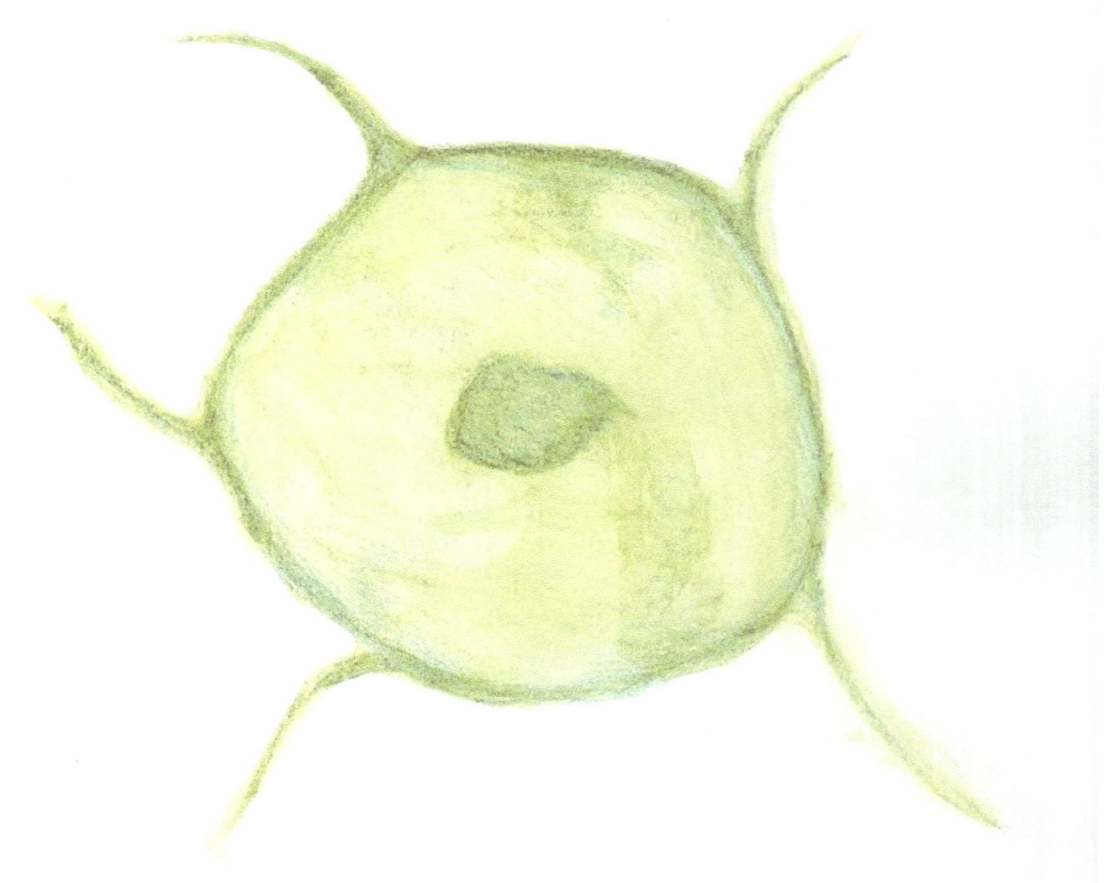

This is what a cell looks like
under a microscope.

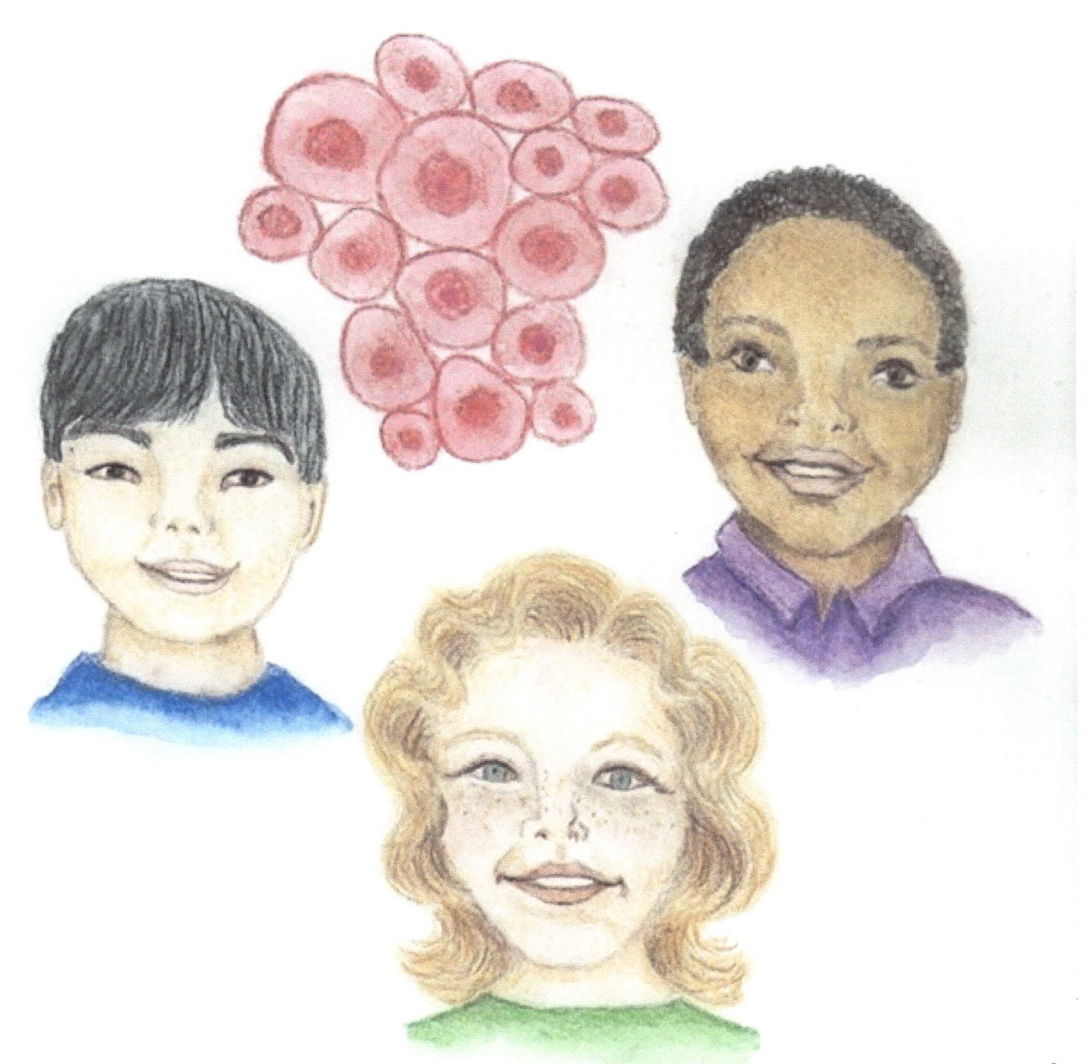

When my cells are happy, my brain
and body work better.

It makes my body happy, and it makes me happy.

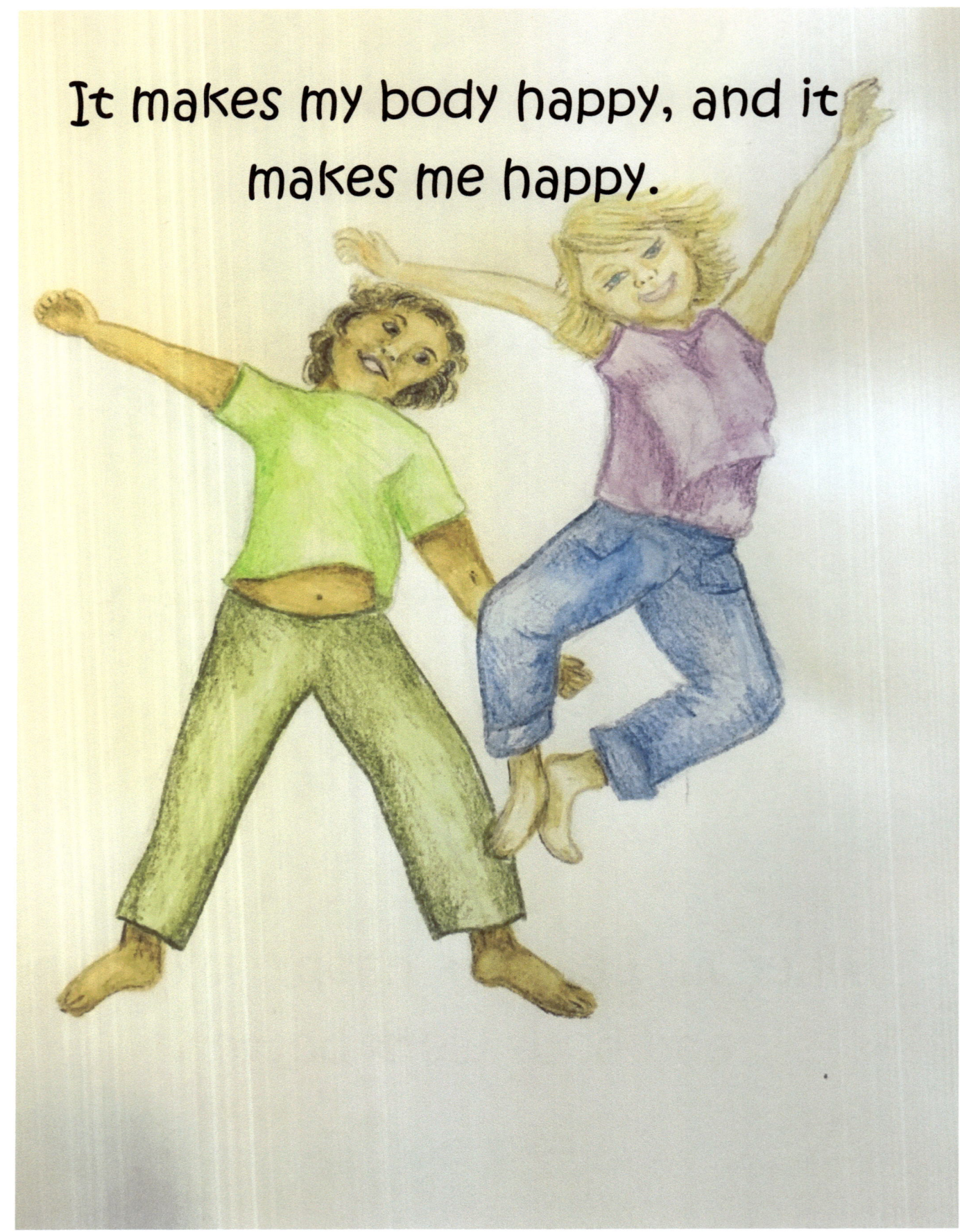

My cells are happy when...

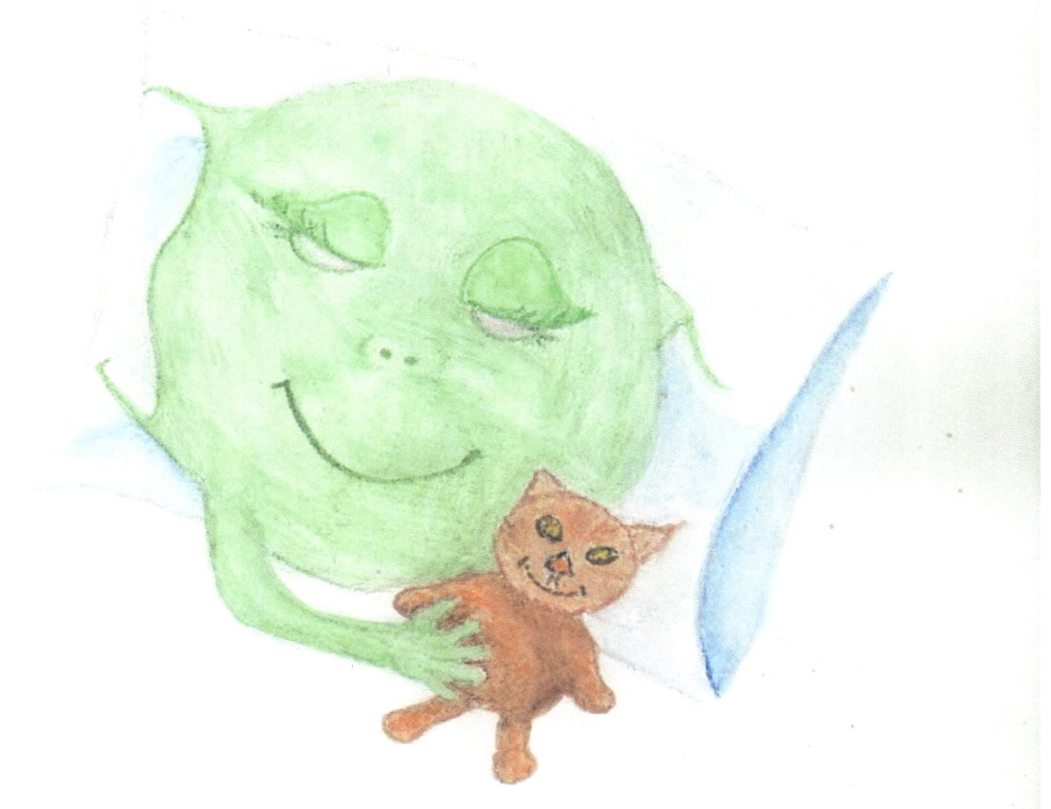

I get plenty of sleep.

My cells are happy when...

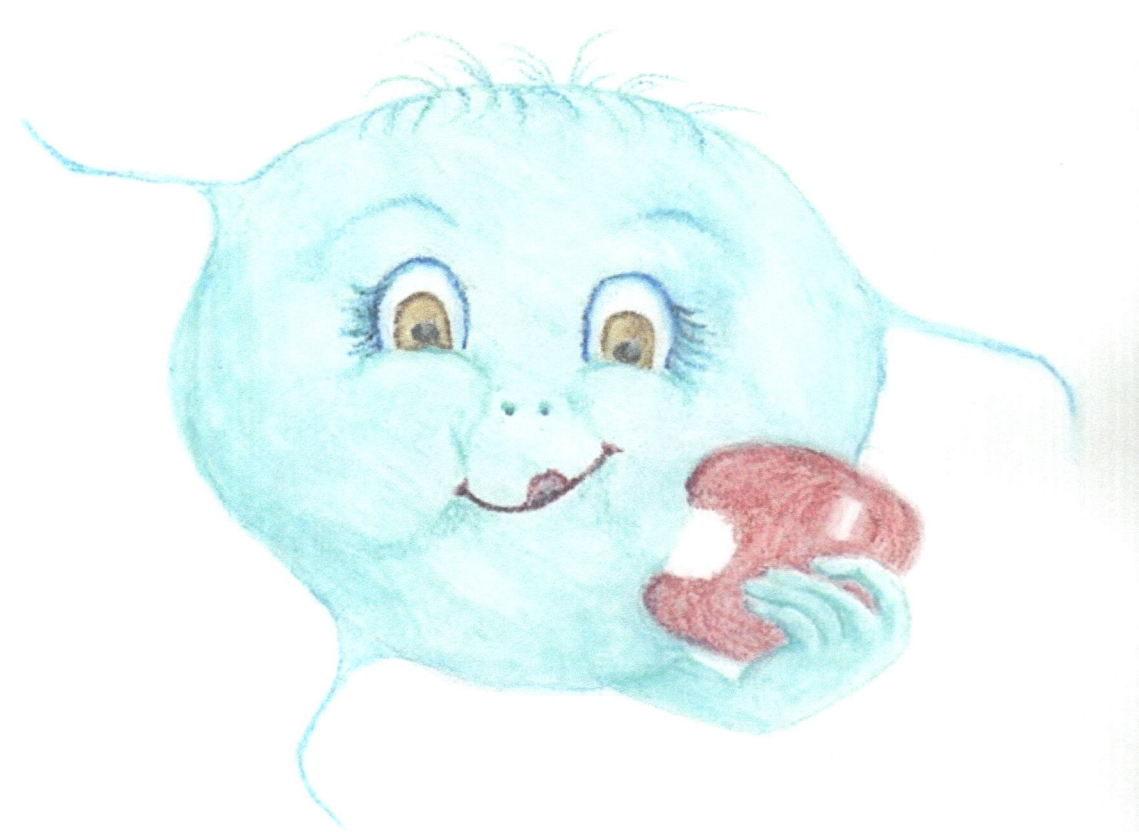

I eat food that is good for me.

My cells are happy when...

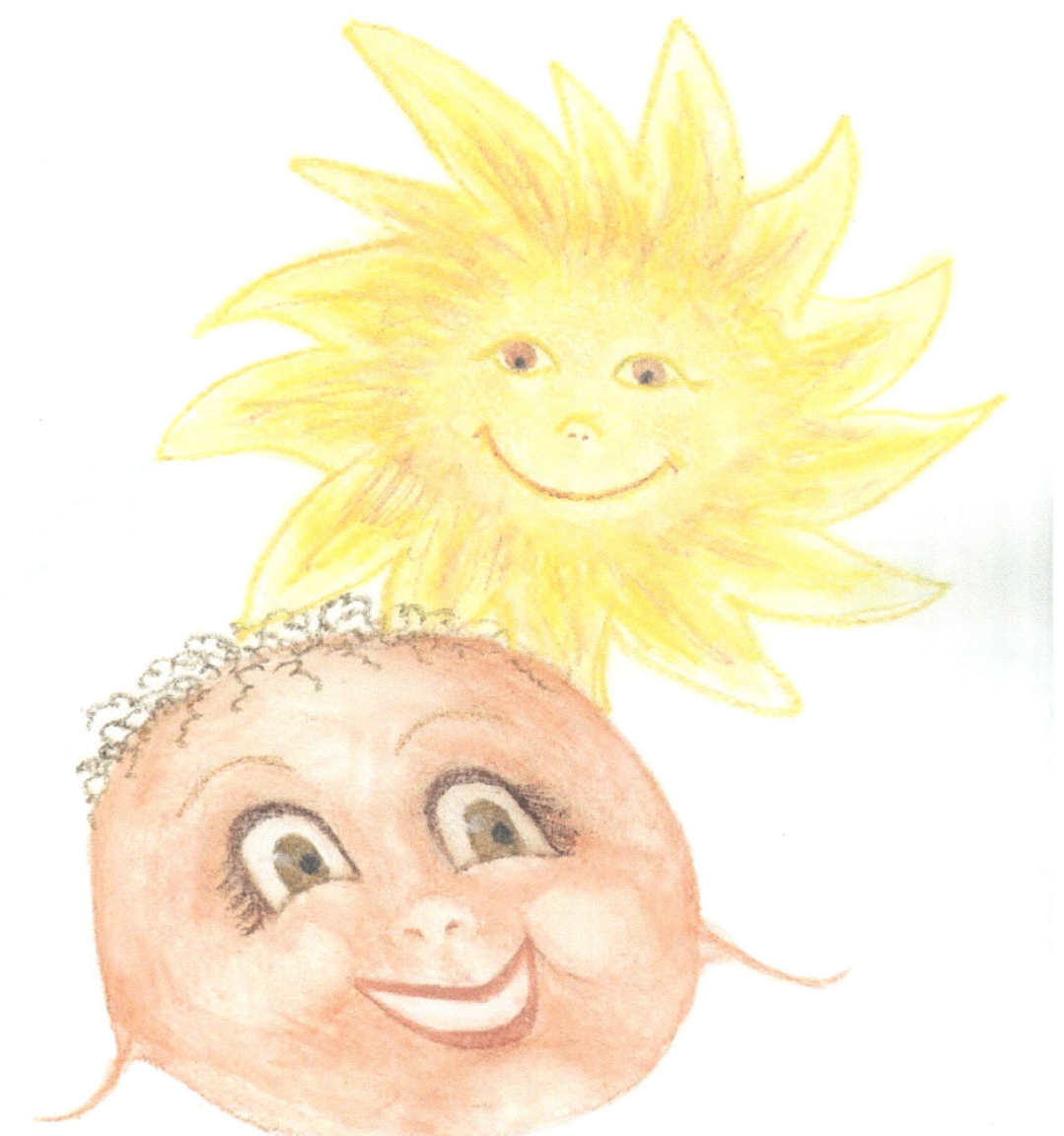

I spend time outside in the sun and fresh air.

My cells are happy when...

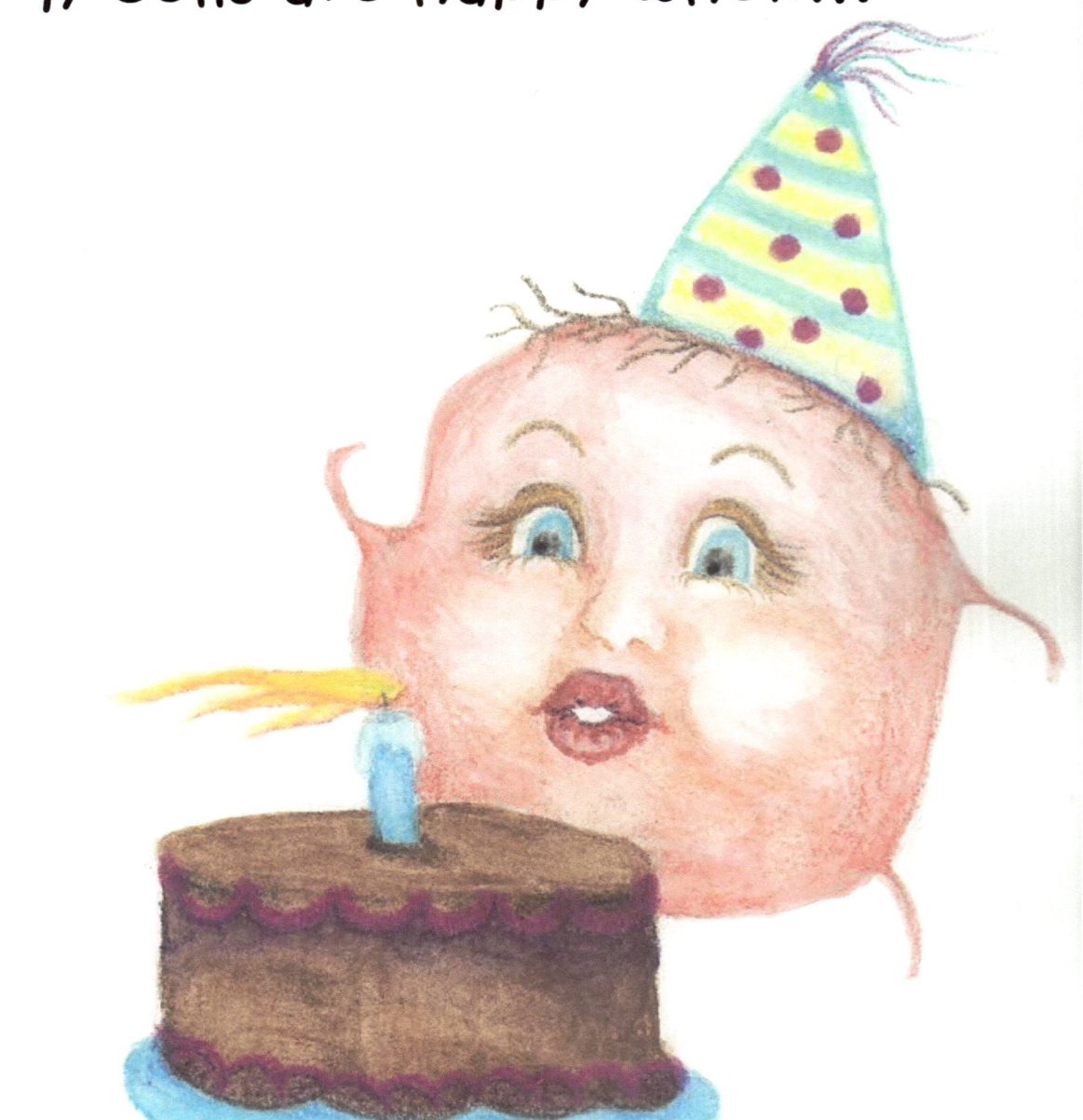

I celebrate my birthday!

My cells are happy when...

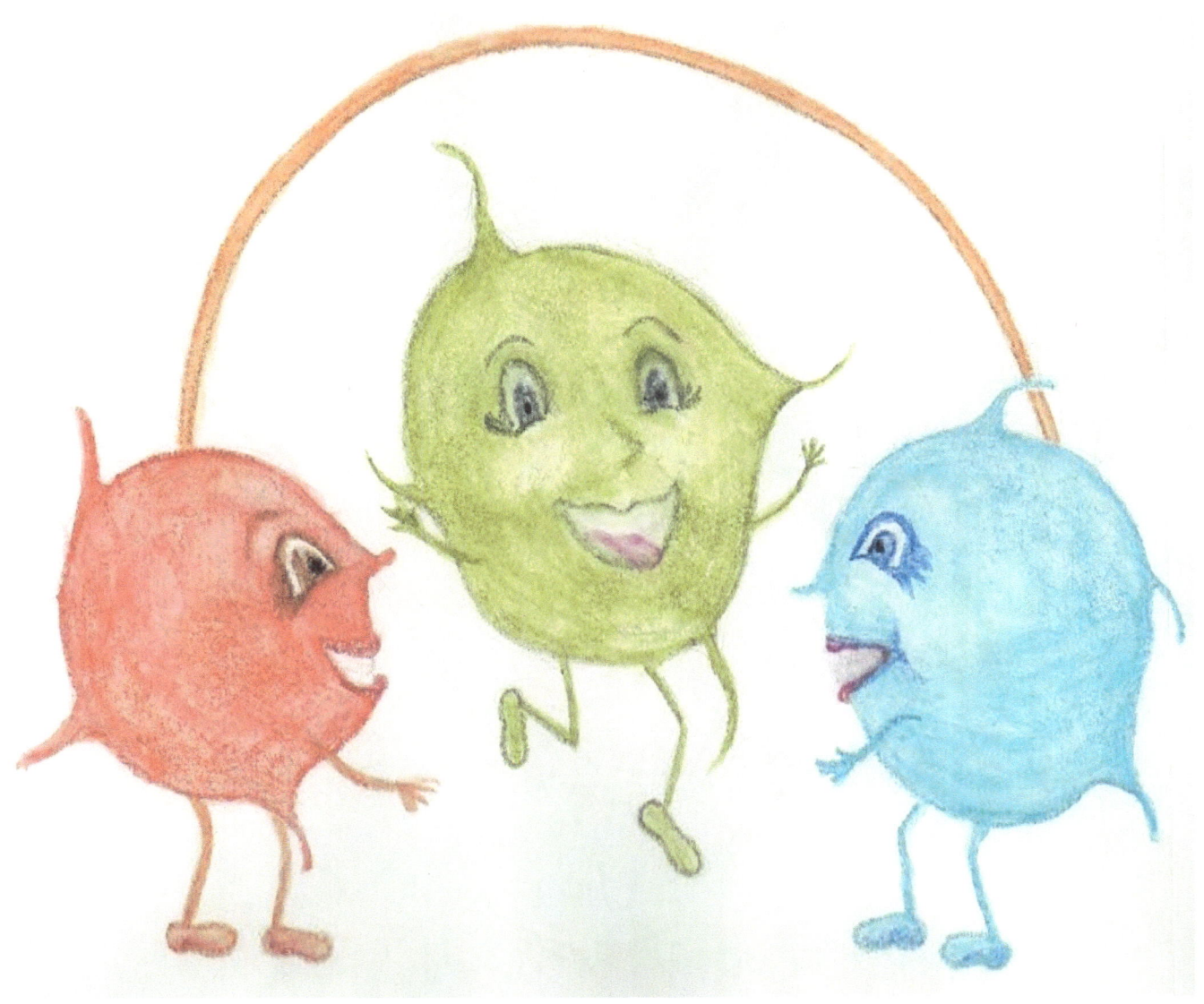

I play outside with my friends.

My cells are happy when...

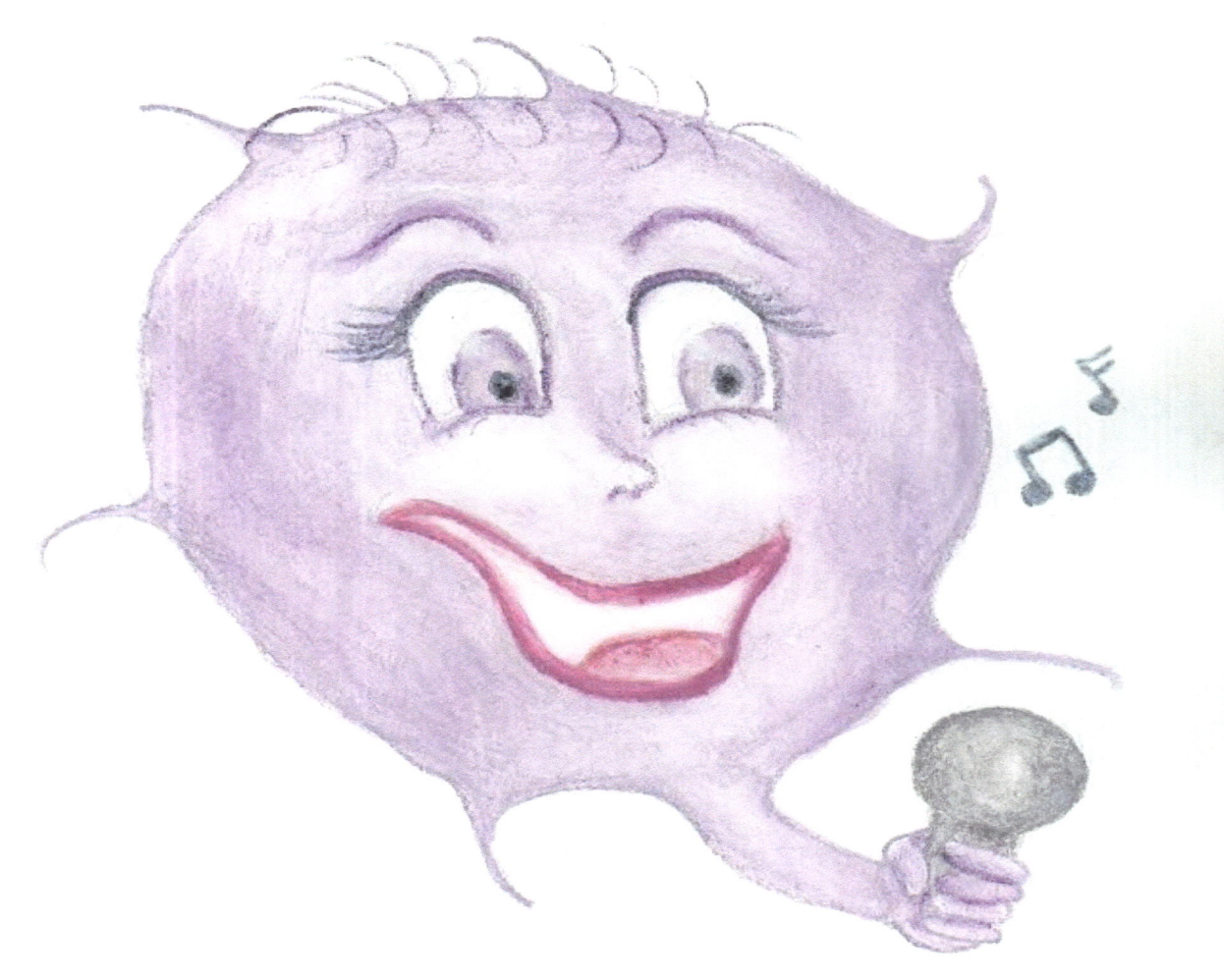

I sing happy songs.

My cells are happy when...

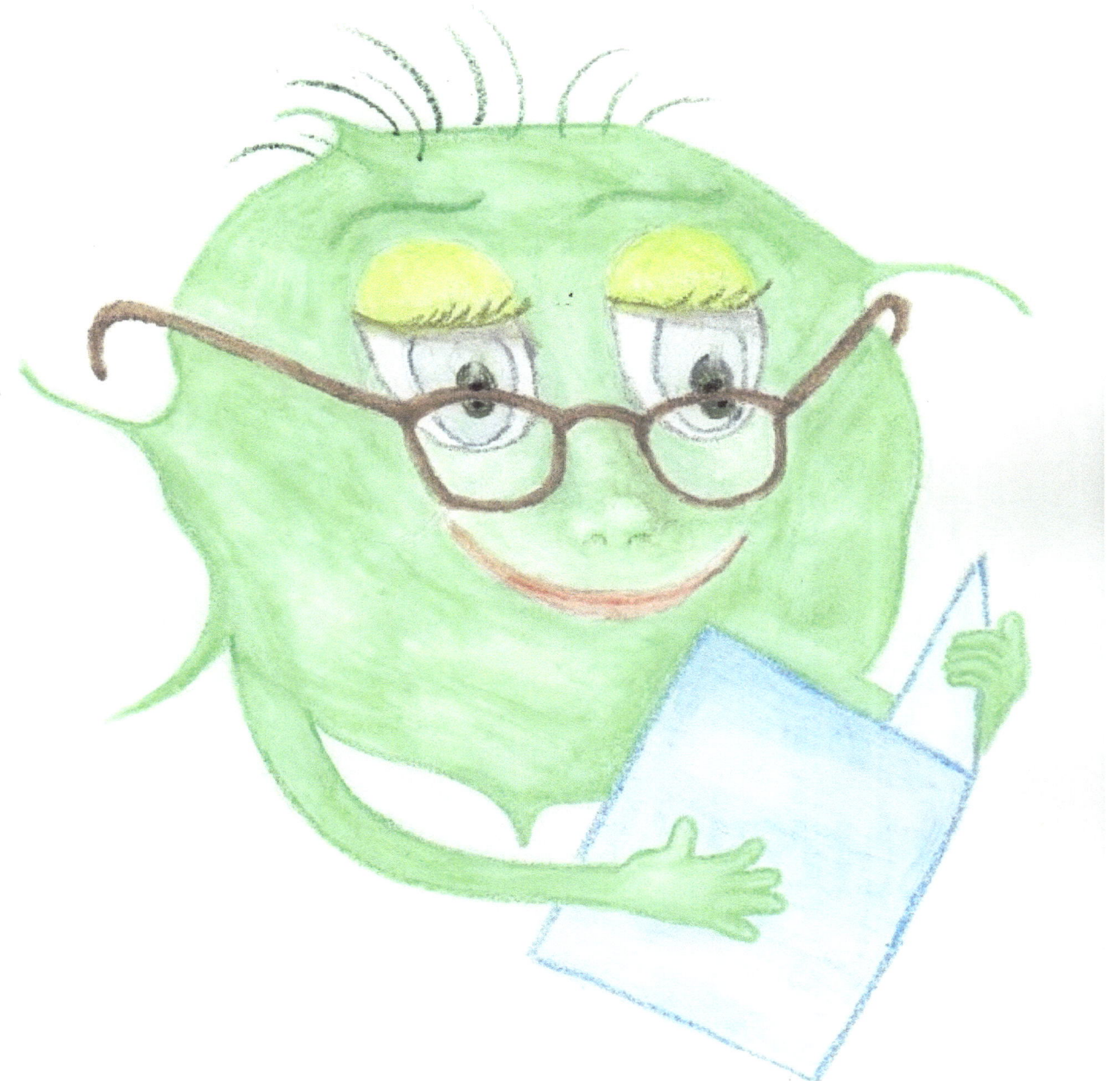

I read a good book.

My cells are happy when...

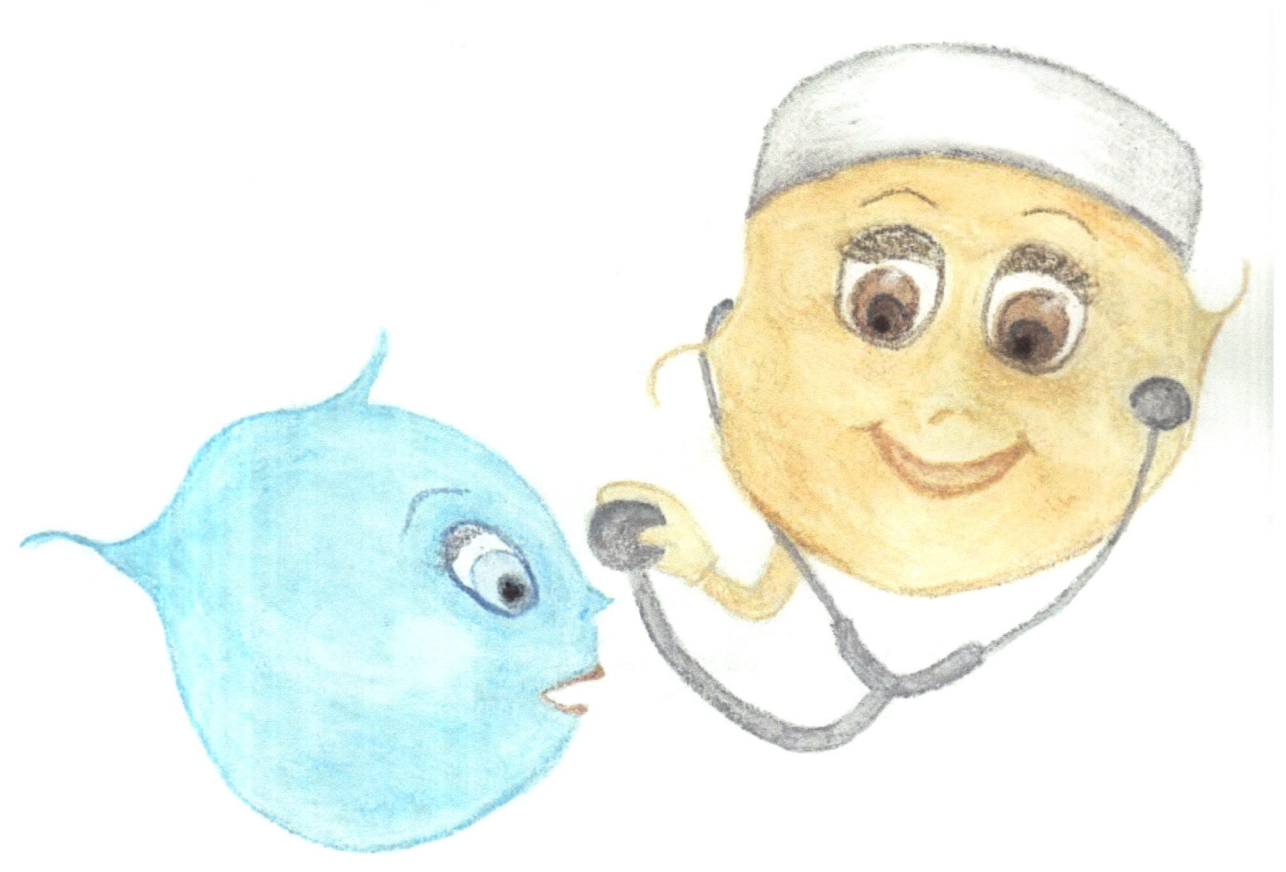

I go to the doctor for a checkup.

My cells are happy when...

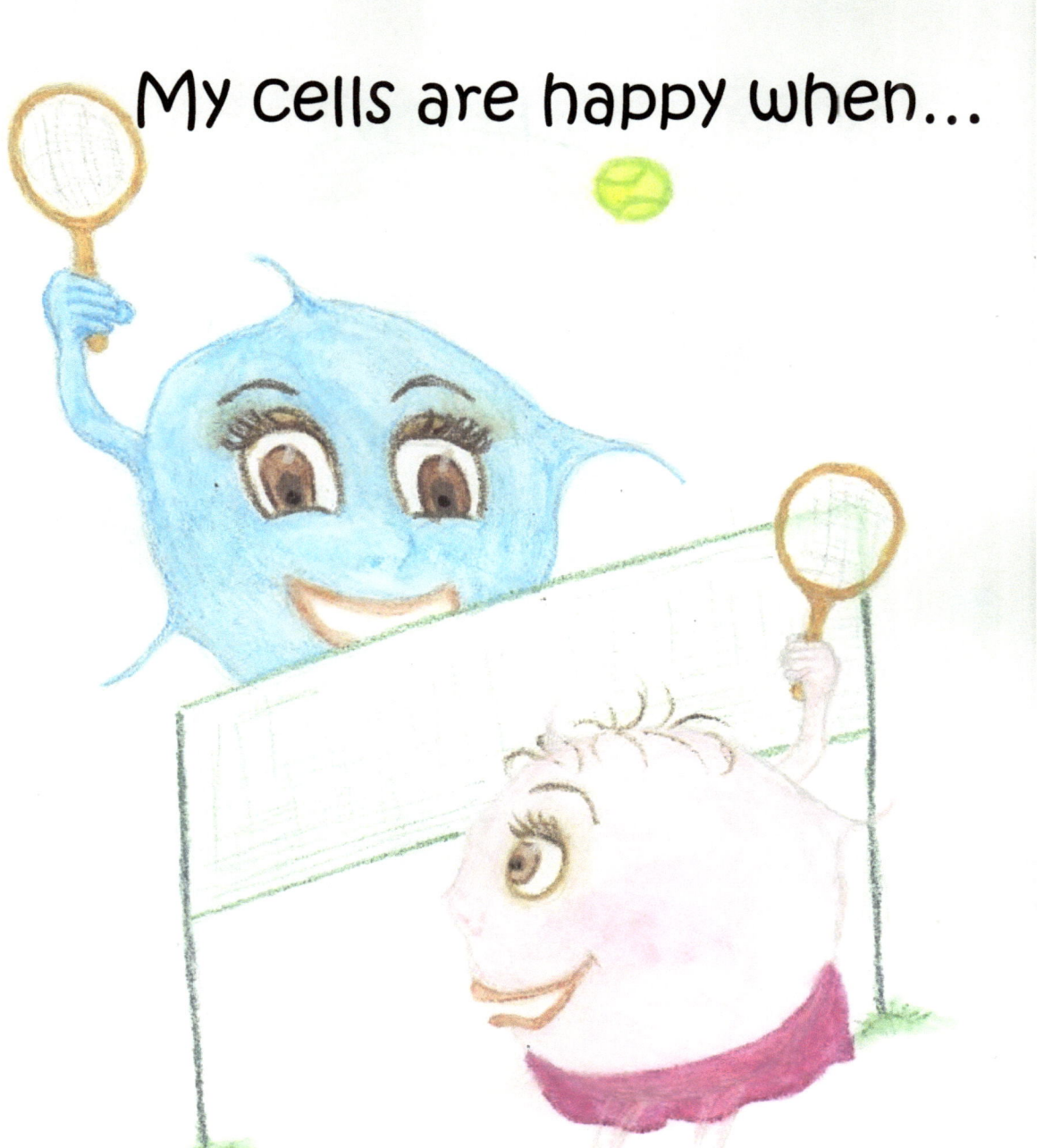

I play sports with my friends.

My cells are happy when...

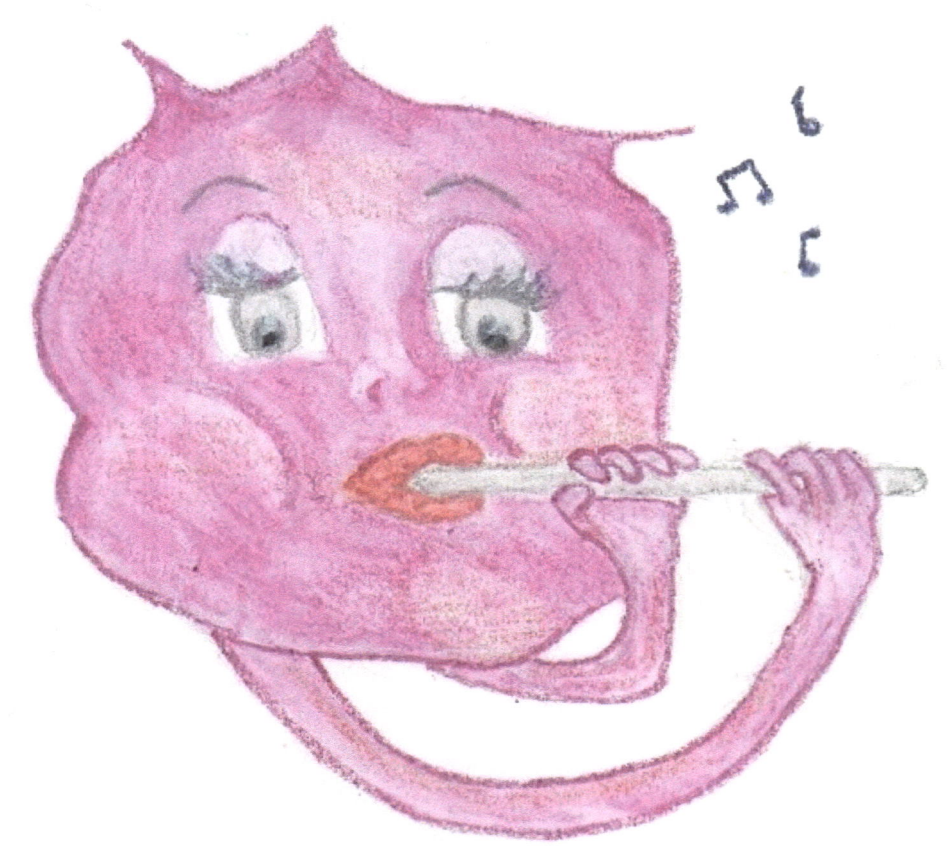

I play musical instruments.

My cells are happy when...

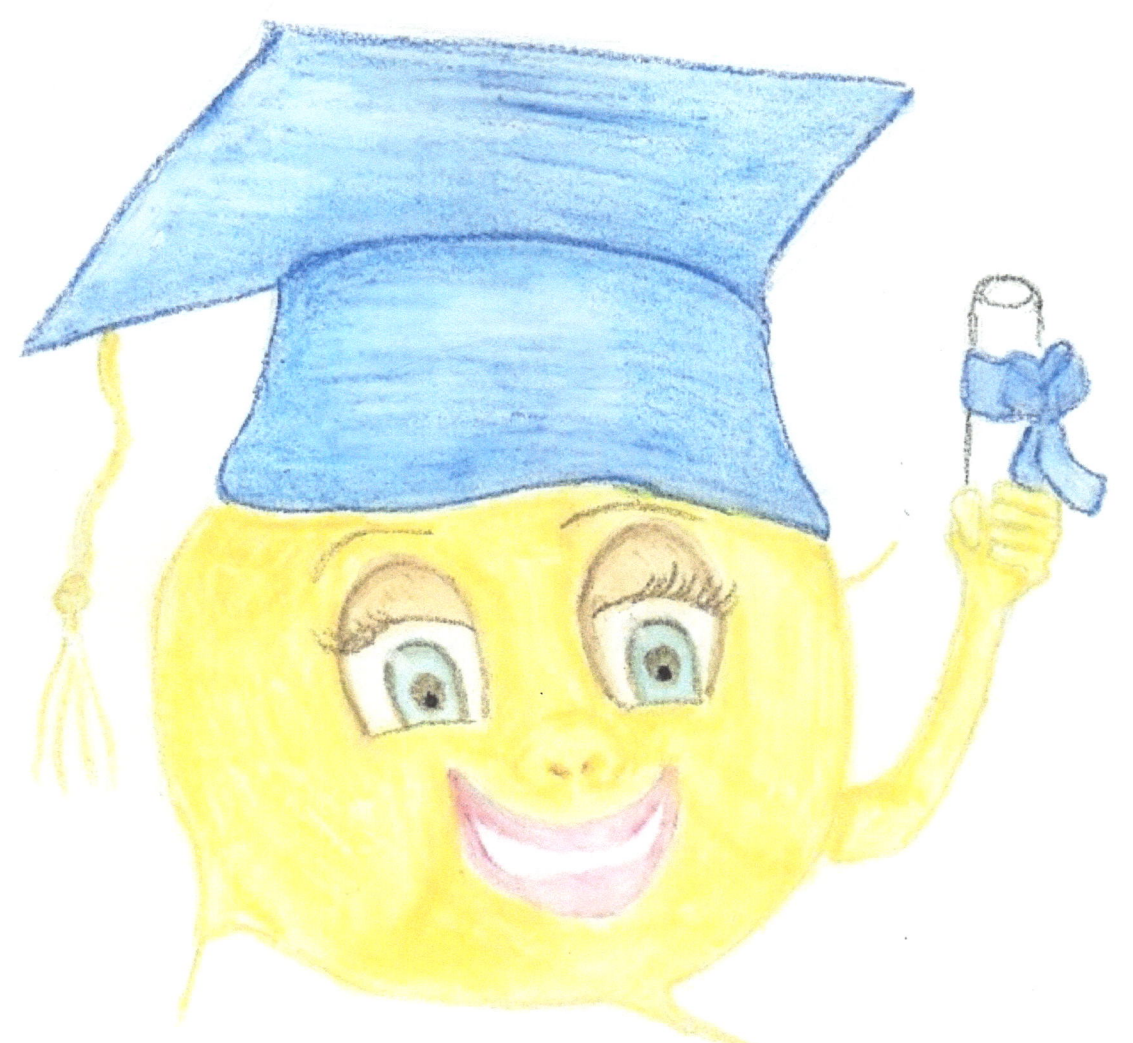

I go to school and learn
new things.

My cells are happy when...

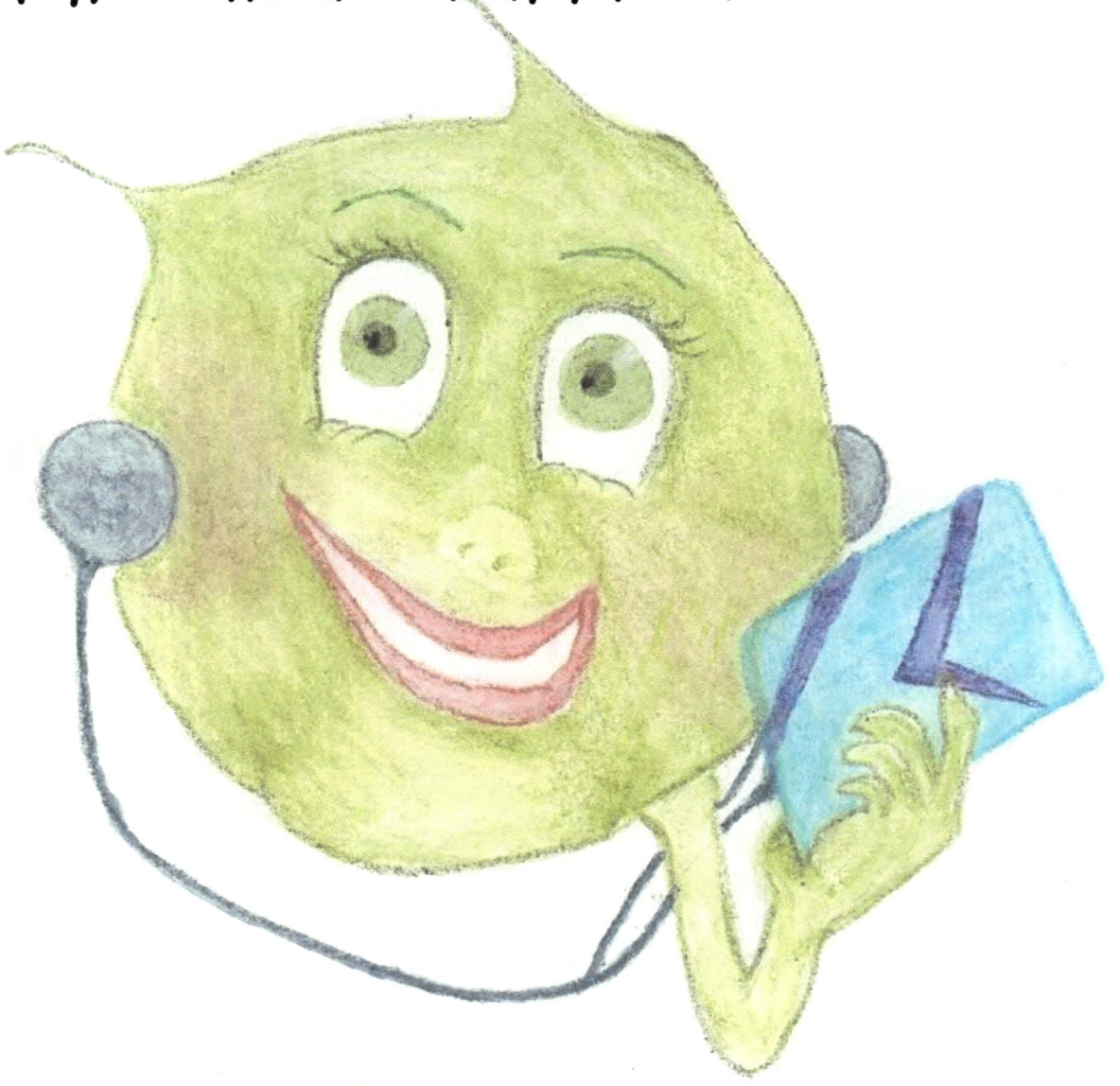

I listen to good music.

My cells are happy when...

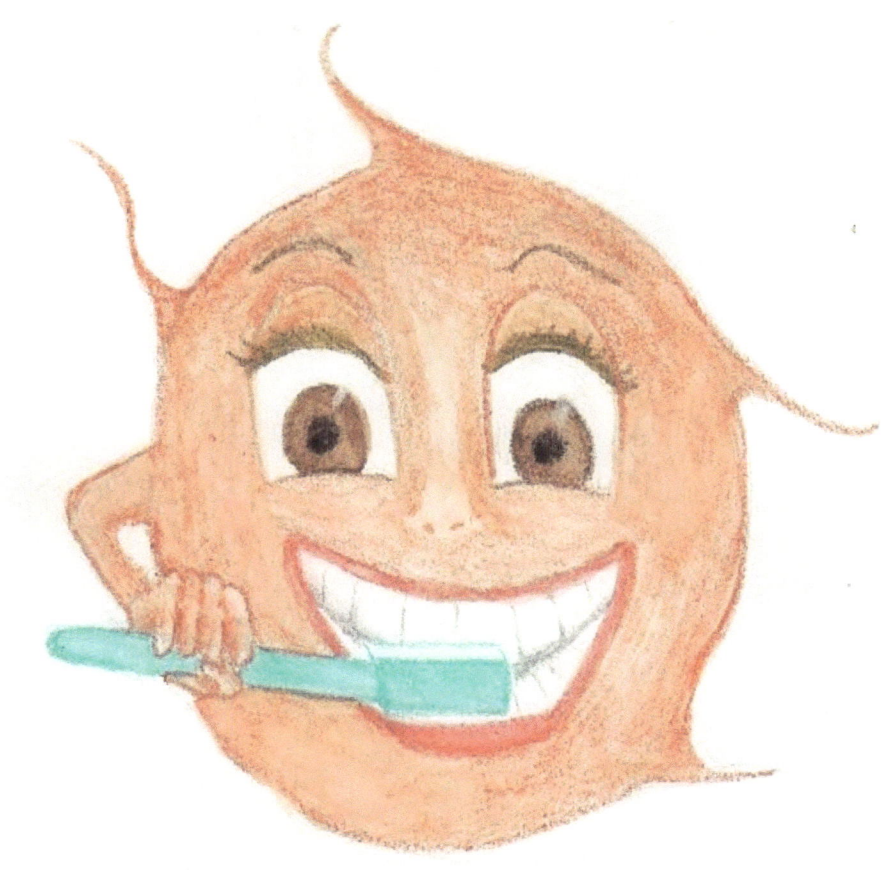

I floss and brush my teeth.

My cells are happy when...

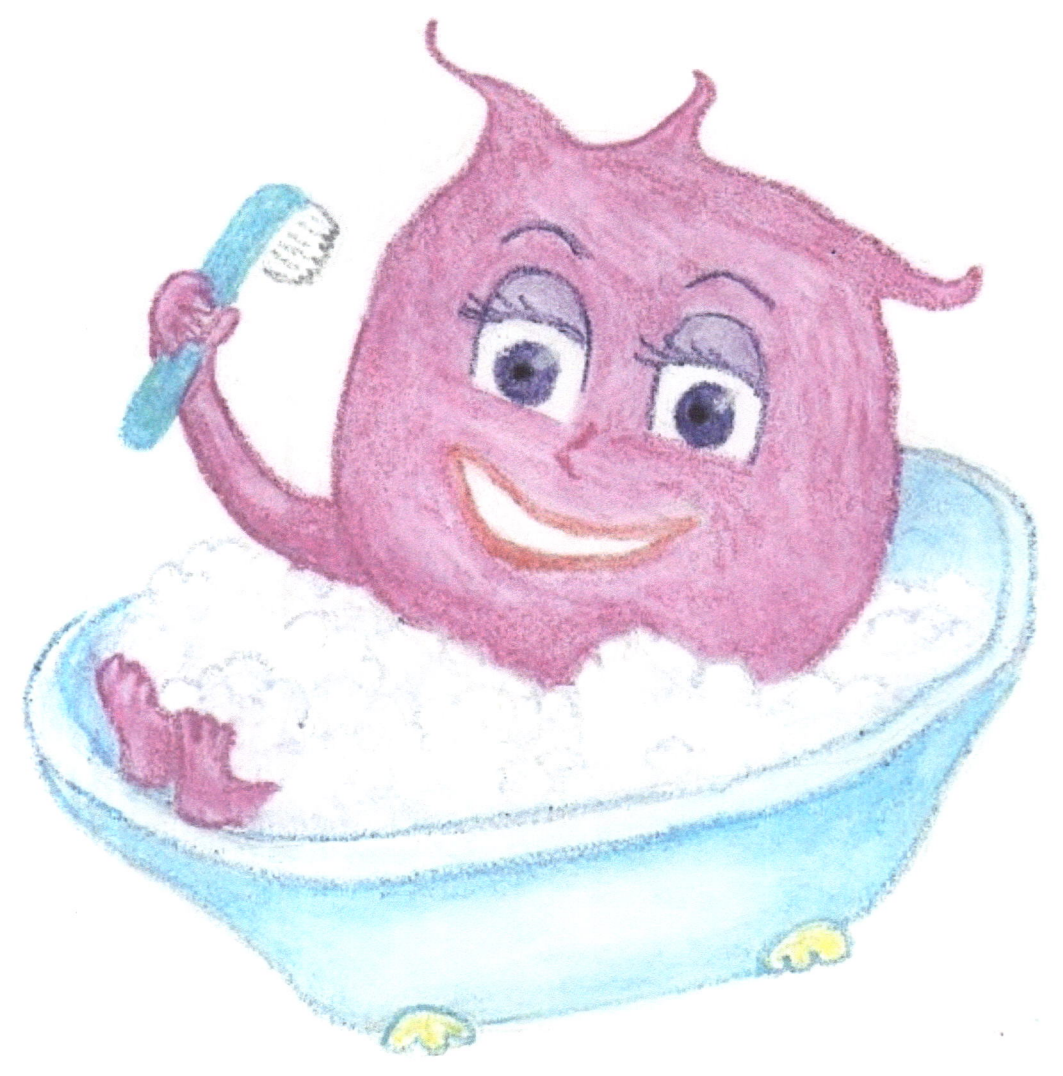

I take a bath.

My cells are happy when...

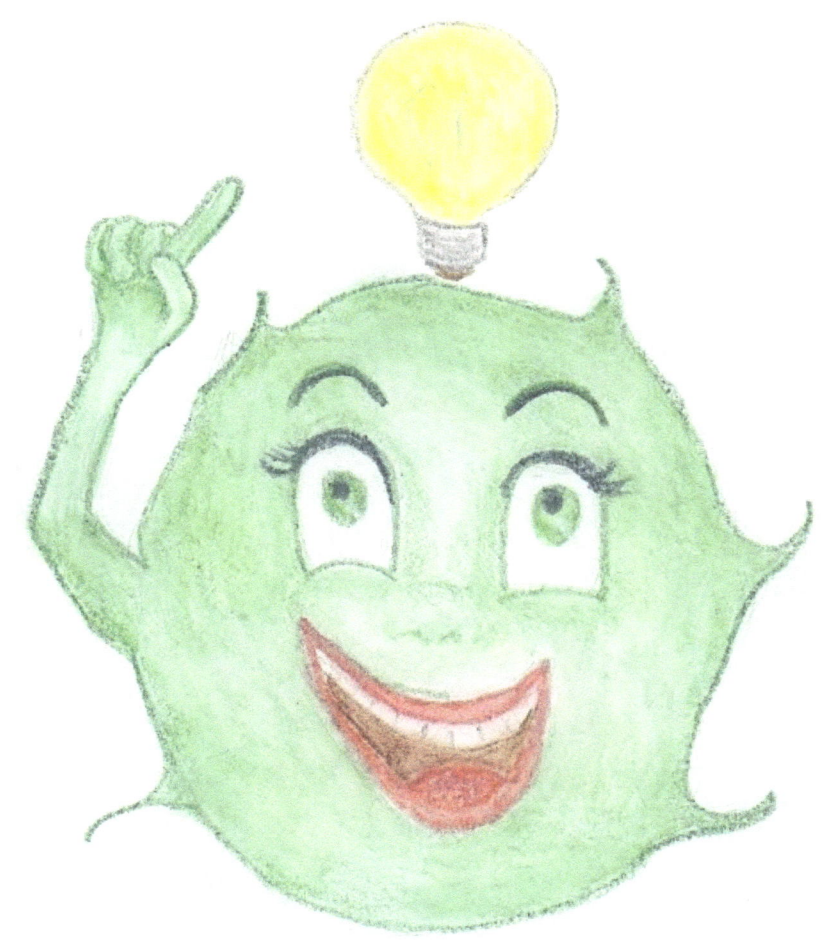

I think of new ideas.

My cells are happy when...

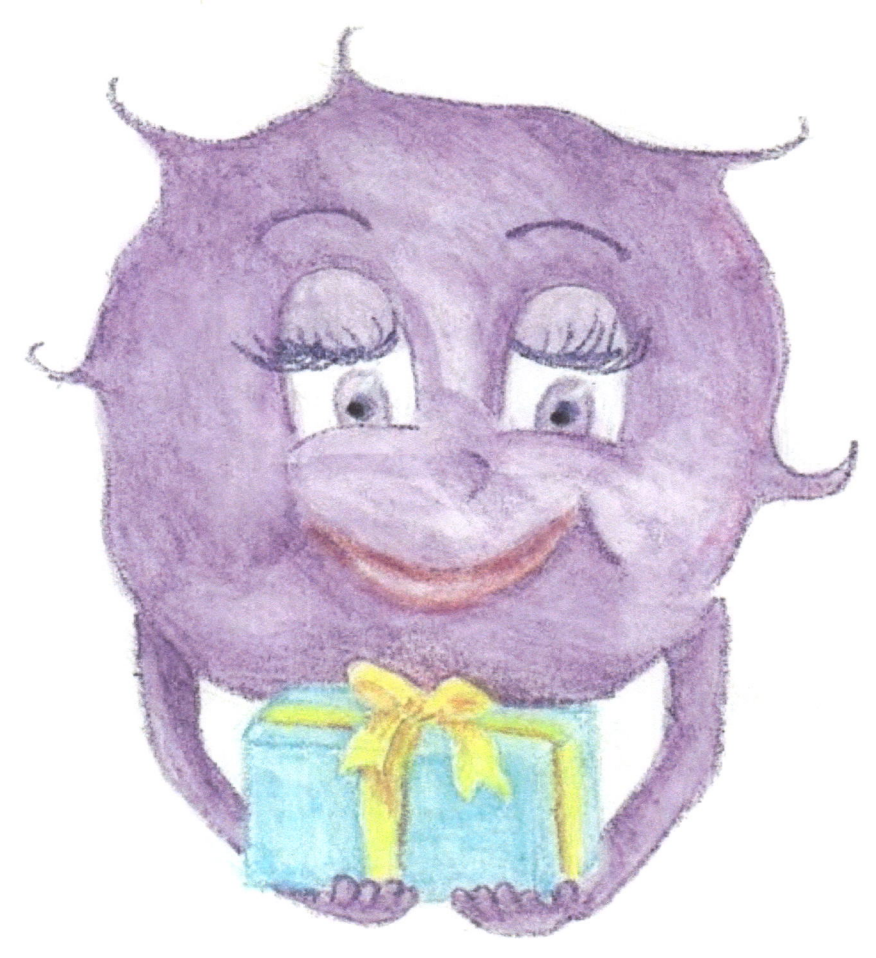

I give to others.

My cells are happy when...

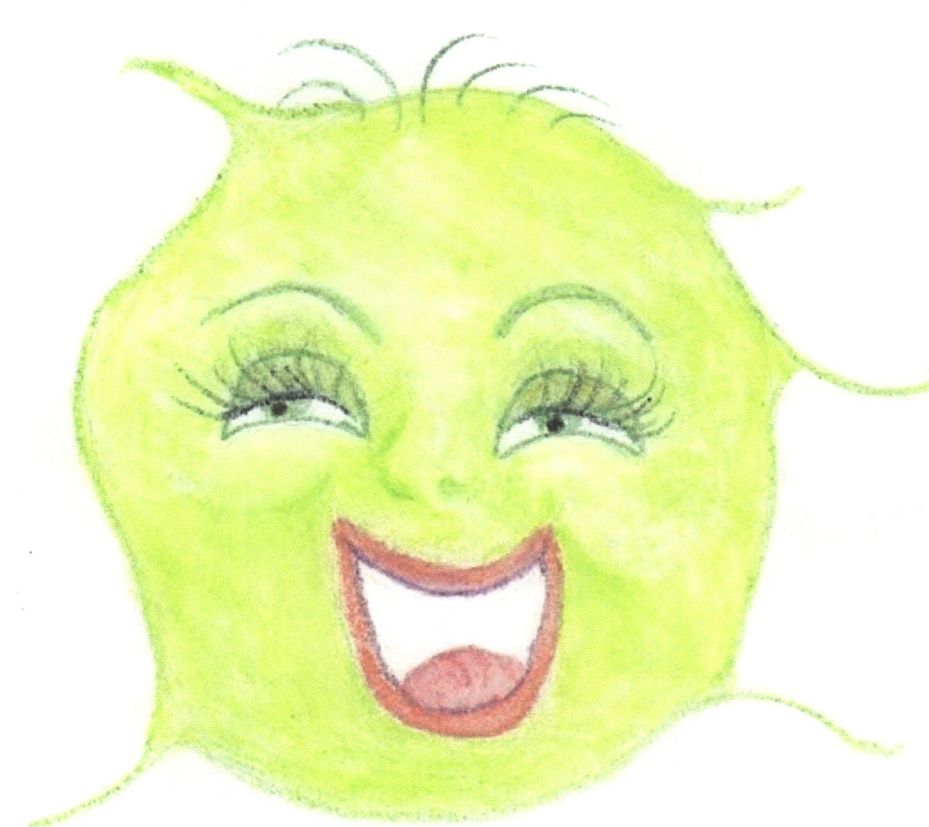

I laugh out loud. LOL!

My cells are happy when...

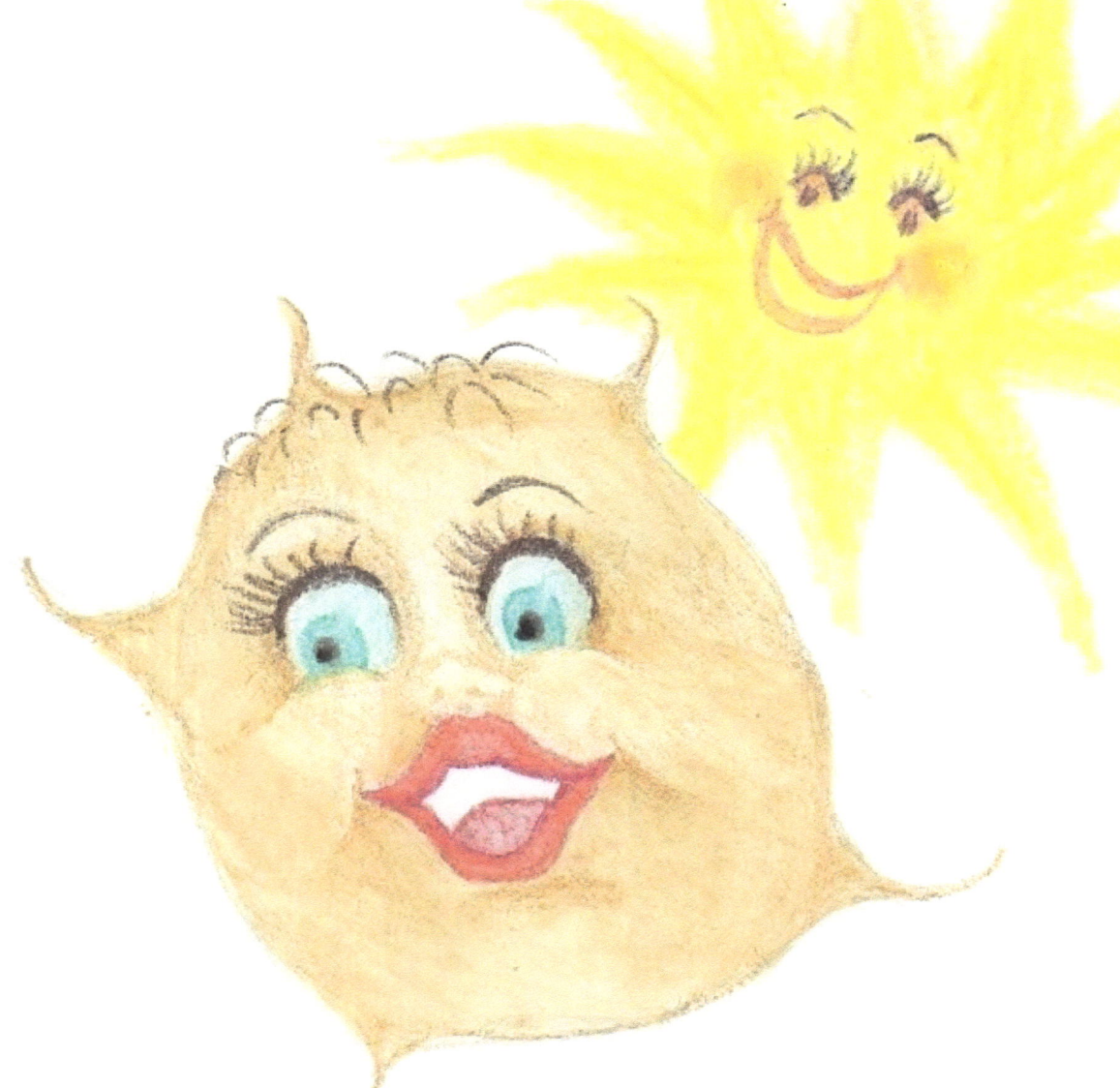

I decide to have a
happy day!

I hope your cells are
as happy as mine.

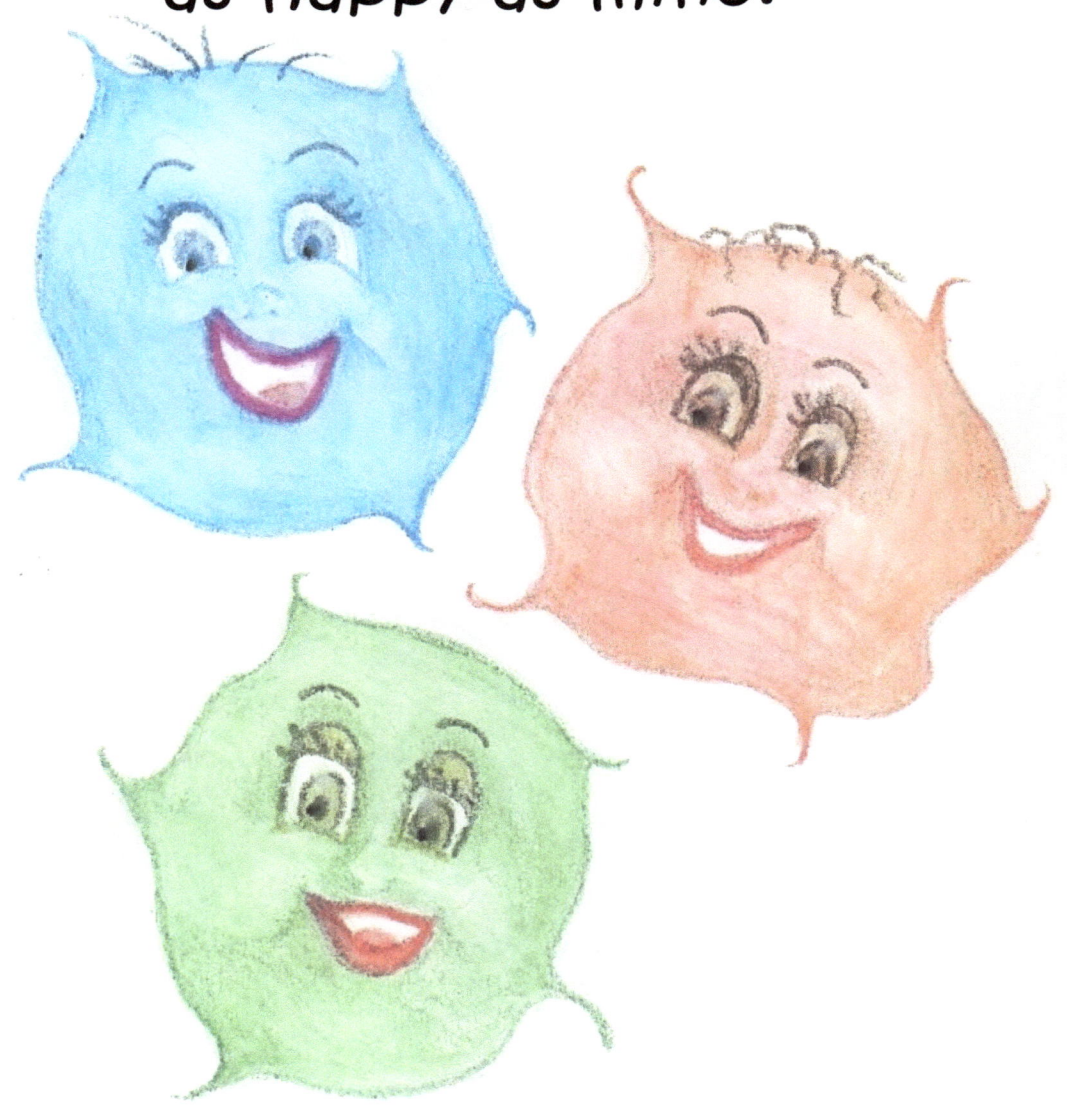

Have a happy day!